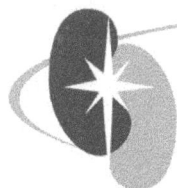

Renal Diet HQ IQ
Teaching You To Master Your Health

Exercising With Chronic Kidney Disease: Solutions to an Active Lifestyle

By Mathea Ford, RD/LD

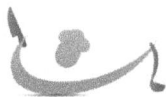

RENALDIET
HEADQUARTERS
BY HEALTHY DIET MENUS FOR YOU

Purpose and Introduction

What I have found through the emails and requests of my readers is that it is difficult to find information about a pre-dialysis kidney diet that is actionable. I want you to know that is what I intend to provide in all my books. You can take these recipes from our website and information to create meals that you and your family will enjoy and they all fit a stage 2 – 5 kidney disease patient.

I wrote this book with you in mind: the person with kidney problems who does not know where to start or can't seem to get the answers that you need from other sources. This book will provide information that is applicable to a predialysis kidney disease diet.

Who am I? I am a registered dietitian in the USA who has been working with kidney patients for my entire 15 + years of experience. Find all my books on Amazon on my author page: http://www.amazon.com/Mathea-Ford/e/B008E1E7IS/

My goals are simple – to give some answers and to create an understanding of what is typical. In this series of 12 books, I will take you through the different parts of being a person with pre-dialysis kidney disease. It will not necessarily be what happens in your case, as everyone is an individual. I may simplify things in an effort to write them so that I feel you can learn the most from the information. This may mean that I don't say the exact things that your doctor would say. If you don't understand, please ask your doctor.

I want you to know, I am not a medical doctor and I am not aware of your particular condition. Information in this book is current as of publication, but may or may not have changed. This book is not meant to substitute for medical treatment for you, your friends, your caregivers, or your family members. You should not base treatment decisions solely on what is contained in this book. Develop your treatment plan with your doctors, nurses and the other medical professionals on your team. I recommend that you double-check any information with your medical team to verify if it applies to you.

In other words, I am not responsible for your medical care. I am providing this book for information and entertainment purposes, not medical diagnoses. Please consult with your doctor about any questions that you have about your particular case.

Table of Contents

Introduction

For years it has been shown that regular physical activity is advantageous on many levels and can have a range of benefits. However, it is becoming increasingly clear that for individuals who suffer from chronic kidney disease (CKD), exercising may be even more important, even to those in end-stage renal disease. Studies have shown that regular exercise can increase oxygen levels and improve blood pressure, cholesterol, and mental health. Resistance and aerobic exercise programs can be beneficial to both patients who are on dialysis and those who are pre-dialysis. However, the exercise programs should be started at fairly low intensity levels and progressed slowly and as tolerated to avoid injury and discomfort.

In many instances, individuals with CKD suffer from complications that are associated with CKD but not actually kidney-related, such as cardiovascular disease, diabetes, anemia, and high blood pressure. In fact, heart disease accounts for more than half of all deaths among those with kidney failure. Regular exercise can help decrease the risk of developing cardiovascular disease or complications.

There are many other benefits to starting a regular exercise program while battling CKD. Regular exercise, for instance, can help battle fatigue which is one of the most common complications of CKD. It can also help fight off the symptoms of depression and anxiety. Strength training involves strengthening your muscles using weights or your own body's resistance and can be instrumental in enabling you to perform the activities that you enjoy doing. This can help you lead a more active lifestyle and make it possible for you to be less dependent on those around you. Strength training can also help increase your stamina and endurance as well. This is good for your mental, as well as your physical, health.

The good news is that you don't even have to exercise a lot in order to see benefits of exercise. The advantages come from frequency and not so much from duration. In fact, exercising 20-30 minutes per day 3-5 times per week is enough for most people to see a real difference in both their physical and mental health. In the following book we'll discuss some of the benefits of regular exercise as well as what types of exercises are most advantageous to those individuals who are currently suffering from chronic kidney disease.

Fatigue and Chronic Kidney Disease

The number one complication of chronic kidney disease is fatigue. Most people with CKD do frequently feel tired and this is usually related to anemia. Fatigue can also result from other causes, such as depression, or even inactivity. It's possible for anemia to develop in any stage of kidney disease and get worse as renal disease progresses.

How anemia is related to chronic kidney disease

Anemia occurs when your body doesn't make enough red blood cells which carry oxygen to all the cells in your body. Oxygen is used to change the food that we consume into energy. If we don't have enough red blood cells then we don't have enough oxygen. Without enough oxygen, our tissues and organs have less energy. This can make you feel tired. Some of the symptoms of anemia can include:

- Weakness
- Fatigue
- Dizziness
- Paleness
- Confusion

If anemia goes untreated then your major organs can be affected. Chronic kidney disease is often associated with anemia because renal disease can cause low levels of erythropoietin (a hormone) and/or iron in the body. Healthy kidneys produce erythropoietin. When the body senses that oxygen levels are low, it tells the kidneys to release erythropoietin. Erythropoietin lets your bone marrow know to make more red blood cells which means that more oxygen can be transported in the bloodstream. If the kidneys are damaged, though, they might not make enough erythropoietin.

Foods that are rich in protein carry iron and this helps make hemoglobin. Hemoglobin is a protein in the red blood cells that carries oxygen. One the main sources of iron is red meat. However, most individuals in stage 3-4 of kidney disease are suggested to reduce the amount of protein they eat, so they may not get enough iron from their diets.

Eventually, waste in the bloodstream can accumulate. This can build up and also affect red blood cells. Although healthy kidneys are able to filter toxins from the bloodstream kidneys that are affected with chronic kidney disease have a reduced capacity to filter blood. As a result, the waste remains in the bloodstream. Here it can stay and even cut down the duration of the life of the red blood cells.

Depression

Depression is also very common with chronic kidney disease and can make you feel tired as well. Depression is not the same as feeling "sad about something" It can develop over a period of weeks, months, and even years. It can affect every part of your life, including your eating and sleeping patterns.

Like many other aspects of your health, a professional should treat depression. It should be taken seriously and isn't an indication that you are doing something wrong or that there is a flaw in your character or that you aren't trying hard enough. Some of the most common signs of depression include:

- Constant sadness
- Difficulty making decisions
- Lack of interest in things that used to make you happy
- Sleeping more or less than usual
- Irritability
- Feeling tired all the time

- Lack of appetite
- Forgetfulness
- Regular thoughts of death and/or suicide

It is important to talk to your physician if you have experienced any symptoms that might be associated with depression. They will be able to determine if the symptoms are associated with depression or something else and set you down the right path to treatment.

Lack of Sleep

One of the biggest causes of being tired during the day can be due to your overall sleeping patterns. If your sleeping patterns get disrupted then it can make it difficult for you to enjoy a good night's rest. For instance, napping during the day can make it challenging to sleep during the night and eventually lead to insomnia.

Developing a good sleeping routine is essential when it comes to fighting fatigue. This might mean avoiding long naps during the day, getting up early in the mornings rather than sleeping late into the day, and going to bed at the same time every night. However, what works for some people might not necessarily work for you. You might discover, for instance, that you actually need a short one hour nap during the afternoon in order to be able to sleep well at night. You should just do what is right for you and not worry that it's right or wrong as long as you are not experiencing other problems.

Other causes of tiredness could be physical or medical, such as pain or even sleep apnea. Sleep apnea is a disruption in breathing during sleep. Symptoms can include snoring and actually the stopping of breathing. Many people with sleep apnea wake up from a restless night's sleep feeling tired and fatigued.

If you experience pain throughout the day, you might also have trouble sleeping at night. Pain can take a physical toll on the body which can, in turn, make you feel tired and restless and make it difficult for your body to relax at night.

Lack of Exercise

It might sound ironic, but sometimes lack of activity can actually make you tired. Sometimes your body can get into an inactivity cycle: the more inactive you are, the more fatigued you become. You don't have the energy to exercise but you become tired because you haven't exercised.

Regular physical activity can actually boost your energy levels and increase your stamina so that you don't feel as fatigued as often. Over time, it will become increasingly easier to have the energy you need to exercise as well as to perform the activities that you enjoy. In fact, the increased amount of energy is one of the main benefits that most people enjoy from exercising since fatigue is one of the most crippling complications from chronic kidney disease.

The Benefits of Exercise

Not only can regular exercise help control fatigue, a regular physical exercise program, when integrated into your total treatment plan, can have positive benefits for your overall health. Some of the benefits that you might experience can include improved muscle strength, physical capacity, weight loss, and lower cholesterol levels. Long-term effects might include such things as reduced risk of cardiac disease.

It is important not to overlook the psychological benefits of exercise, too. Chronic kidney disease can have psychological ramifications such as depression, stress, and anxiety. However, regular exercise can improve self-esteem and create a sense of independence which may help control depression and anxiety.

Battling Inflammation

Many individuals suffering from chronic kidney disease have ongoing elevations of inflammation. Inflammation is generally associated with malnutrition and muscle wasting and is seen a lot in chronic kidney disease patients because of the dietary restrictions related to protein.

Inflammation occurs when white blood cells work to protect the body from infective substances like viruses and bacteria. Acute inflammation can last for several days but generally ends once whatever has caused the inflammation has been cleared up. Chronic inflammation, however, happens over a longer period of time and may never really go away.

Although inflammation is technically the body's natural defense when it's under attack, it can also happen when there isn't anything to fight off. Individuals with CKD can experience chronic inflammation which can cause cardiovascular disease and an increased rate of death.

Inflammation can be caused by:

- Malnutrition
- Obesity
- Vascular access infection
- Inactivity
- Insomnia
- Infections
- Gum disease
- Foot ulcer
- Anemia
- Uremia
- A non-functional kidney

Research has shown that an increase in regular physical exercise over a prolonged period of time may help reduce inflammation.

Live Longer

Lack of physical activity has actually been linked to an increased risk of chronic kidney disease. In addition, inactive chronic kidney disease patients are at an additional increased risk of a shorter lifespan whereas those who exercise at least 4-5 times per week have a significantly lower rate of dying due to a kidney disease related illness.

According to a study done by the University of Utah in Salt Lake City, those who got the recommended amount of weekly exercise were 56% less likely to die through seven years of follow-up than those who did not exercise at all. Those who exercised, but at less than the recommended level of activity, were still 42% less likely to die during follow-up than sedentary patients. The study noted that most patients with chronic kidney disease pass away before developing end-stage renal disease, but the current focus for clinicians is on slowing the disease progression. However, one measure that may be helpful in improving survival in these patients is increasing exercise.

More Benefits

Additional benefits that can be realized from regular exercise can include:

- Improved muscle functioning
- Improved blood pressure control
- Better muscle strength
- Lower cholesterol levels
- Better quality of sleep
- Weight loss
- Better able to complete activities of daily living

Before you start

One of the first things you'll want to do before embarking upon an exercise program is consult with your physician. They may recommend you submit yourself to a medical examination, and if need be, even a cardiac exam, before you start any kind of exercise program. As long as your condition is considered stable and your physician thinks you'll benefit from regular exercise, you should be given the go-ahead.

While you are exercising, you will also want to continue to comply with any medication and dietary instructions that you are currently following.

What counts as exercise?

Exercising can be made up of a variety of activities and doesn't just have to mean weight lifting and aerobics.

Stretching

Stretching warms up the muscles by getting the blood circulating throughout the body. You can also do it anywhere without any special workout equipment. You should stretch before exercising and afterward to help you cool down.

Indoor cardio exercises

Cardio exercises mainly benefit the heart. Cardio exercise is good for your heart for several reasons. It is a repetitive, rhythmic exercise that increases your heart rate when you're exercising and requires your body to use more oxygen. The more your heart works, the stronger it becomes and the more efficient it becomes. Like any other muscle in your body and it needs to be exercised. As it is strengthened, your resting heart rate will be reduced and it won't have to work as hard when you're not working out. Your circulation will be improved and your red blood cell capacity will be increased. These carry oxygen through your blood to your different tissues.

Indoor cardio equipment examples can include a treadmill or stationary bike. As an alternative, you can also simply walk or jog in place to get your heart rate up. If your home has a staircase, you can walk up and down the stairs for your cardio workout. If your home doesn't have a staircase, try going to a local indoor mall for a vigorous walk. You may need to walk around the mall a few times to get the most benefit out of your walk.

Weight lifting

Weight lifting might be an indoor exercise that is an option for you. However, if you have an arteriovenous (AV) fistula in your arm for hemodialysis or an abdominal catheter for peritoneal dialysis, you should talk to your doctor before you lift any weights.

Lifting light weights can help you increase your blood flow. It can also help you improve your strength. You can do it in a gym or in your own home, for example, in front of your television while you are sitting down.

Calisthenics

Calisthenics use your body's weight for resistance and help strengthen and improve the body's flexibility. You don't need any special workout equipment for this kind of exercising so you can do it inside. Different kinds include:

- **Crunches**: Stomach crunches are like sit-ups except you only lift your upper back instead of your whole back. This allows you to isolate your ab muscles and give them a workout.
- **Sit-ups**: In sit-ups, you workout your whole back, including your abs and your hips. You generally do these with your knees bent and your elbows locked behind your head.
- **Push-ups**: Push-ups use your own body weight as resistance for strength training exercises. You can stretch in full length for the most resistance and attempt to lift your entire body weight off the ground with your arms. Optionally, you can rest on your knees and push up using your arms, to support yourself until you've gained strength in your upper arms to support your entire weight first.
- **Pull-ups**: Pull-ups are a form of strength-training that involve pulling one's self up using a bar raised above your head. You rely on your upper body strength to support your own body weight.
- **Jumping Jacks:** Jumping jacks are started from a standing position with legs together and arms at the sides. From there, you jump until the legs are apart and the arms are over your head. The movements are done at the same time. Then, you jump back to the original position and repeat quickly. The movements are repeated in secession.

- **Squats:** Squats use your own body weight as resistance and can be done in rapid secession as well. Keeping your back straight, bend your knees until your buttocks nearly touch your heels and hold as long as possible and then stand up. Repeat.

Other activities

Even when you're not actively exercising there are other activities you can do to give your muscles the work out they need to stay flexible and supple. For instance, various chores around the house can keep you up and moving on your feet. Simply sweeping, mopping, and even organizing a room can be enough to get your blood pumping. Other examples of good activities that can be good forms of exercising include:

- Vacuuming
- Laundry
- Cleaning out your dresser drawers or closet
- Dusting
- Moving the furniture around
- Gardening

What Else Can You Gain from an Exercise Program?

In addition to the previous benefits you can gain from incorporating a regular exercise program into your overall treatment plan, there are additional advantages to exercising as well. These include increased core strength, increased endurance, and more flexibility. All of these help improve your overall health as well, but in different ways. It's important to build up to the level needed over time.

Strength training – how to improve your strength and how it's valuable

Studies show that strength training has health benefits that go beyond merely bulking up and strengthening bones. More lean muscle mass may possibly allow kidney dialysis patients to live longer, boost the good kind of cholesterol, offer older individuals better cognitive function, lessen the symptoms of depression, lower the risk of diabetes, and even reduce the swelling and soreness of lymphedema after breast cancer.

Research has shown that moderate to intense strength training can build skeletal muscle and increase bone density which is important, especially as people age since bone density can naturally lessen over time. During strength training exercises, muscles generate more force than they do during endurance exercises and the heart's muscle tissue contracts forcefully to push the blood out. This helps make a stronger heart which results in one that is more efficient at pumping.

Strength training will also help improve the way your body uses the glucose in your blood (your blood sugar levels). This can reduce the risk of diabetes which is important for individuals with CKD. Strength training increases the number of hormones that take glucose out of the blood and move it into the skeletal muscle. This gives the muscles more energy and lowers the general blood-glucose levels. If your glucose levels are uncontrolled because you have diabetes, then you can have kidney damage and that can cause damage to other organs like your heart and eyes.

For those already suffering from CKD, strength training exercises can be extra helpful. In a 2010 study in the Clinical Journal of the American Society of Nephrology it was discovered that those individuals on dialysis who had the leanest muscle mass were 37% less likely to die than those who had the least.

In resistance training, avoid heavy weights since these can increase your blood pressure to unsafe levels for kidney disease. It's safer to use lighter weights and to use proper breathing techniques. When it comes to repetitions and frequency, do 6 - 10 exercises targeting the large muscle groups: legs, abdomen, back, chest and arms. Perform the exercises using free weights or weight machines. Do the resistance training 2-3 times a week. To prevent injury and ensure you get the benefit of the resistance training, don't do these exercises two days in a row. Spread them out a little bit, such as every other day and cycle the muscle groups you train.

5 Ways to Improve Your Strength

1. Take the stairs to strengthen the muscles in your legs.

2. Some cardiovascular exercises such as swimming and biking can also strengthen muscles as well and give you a good workout. Water walking/water aerobics are excellent exercises that can be done in swimming pools and are especially good for those who have problems with their joints. Water walking offers your submerged muscles nearly 14 times the resistance of air yet also offers gentle pressure on them as well.

3. If you're lifting weights, start out slowly and gradually increase your endurance. Even the smallest amount of resistance can help-some people start out with soup cans!

4. Attach ankle weights when you walk for added resistance.

5. Continue to stay hydrated while exercising so that your muscles remain flexible to avoid injury.

4 Exercises to Do At Home

1. Leg Abduction

1. While lying on your side, brace your abdomen.
2. Bend your top knee and place your top foot in front of your bottom knee.
3. Raise your lower leg off the floor. Don't let your trunk bend backward.
4. Keep your core engaged and feel this on the inside of your lower leg. Repeat 10 times, and switch to the other side.

2. Straight Leg Raises

1. Lying flat on your back, hold your core.
2. Bend one leg up at the knee, and keep the other leg straight.
3. Tighten the quad muscle of your straight leg and raise it up off the floor until your thighs are parallel. Hold this position 5 seconds then lower your leg until it almost touches the floor. Repeat 10 times. Switch to the other leg.

3. Heel Step Downs

1. Stand with your feet together, and take a step forward.
2. When your heel hits the floor, keep it from flexing down as you shift your weight forward.
3. Return your foot to the starting position, and repeat on the other side.
4. Perform 10 of these on each side.

4. Side Plank

1. Lie on your side and brace your core muscles.
2. Raise yourself up on the side of one foot and your elbow.
3. Raise your trunk off the floor. Don't let your middle sag. Squeeze your oblique muscles (the muscles that cover the sides of your stomach).
4. Hold for 10-20 seconds. Repeat. Build up to 30-60 seconds over time.

Endurance Training – How To Increase Your Endurance and Why It Matters

Endurance training is beneficial to your heart, lungs and circulation and helps this work more efficiently. For renal patients, walking is considered to be one of the best cardiovascular exercises although, depending on your current mobility level, you might find other activities just as enjoyable. Cardiovascular exercises will help improve your endurance and stamina so that you are able to be active for longer periods of time without becoming tired.

It's important to build up your endurance levels gradually so that you're not overdoing it. You might want to start out with 5 minutes of exercises at a time and build up from there. If you've been inactive for a long time then it's particularly important to start out slowly and gradually increase your level of activity over a period of time. It may take you months to go from a very long-standing inactive lifestyle to participating in regular physical activity. You want to work your way up to a moderate level of exercise that increases your breathing and heart rate but you don't want to do it all at once because that could compromise your health.

You want to try to exercise for at least 20-30 minutes per day several times a week. Exercising any less than that won't give you the results that you are seeking for your cardiovascular and respiratory systems. However, in the beginning exercising for less than this amount of time will help you increase your endurance and build up to the level needed.

By increasing your endurance over time you'll be able to gradually exercise at a pace that is comfortable and healthy to you. The endurance activities shouldn't make you breathe so hard that you're unable to talk. They shouldn't cause you any dizziness or chest pain, either.

Try doing some light activity before and after your exercise sessions in order to warm up and cool down, like a little slow walking. Stretching, too, while your muscles are warm can help. As your body ages it can become more easily dehydrated. As a result, you might need to drink more water than you needed to in the past so it's important to stay hydrated throughout your exercising in order to keep your muscles fluid.

Once your body becomes accustomed to the exercises you've been performing then you can safely increase your activities and the amount of time you spend performing them. First you should gradually increase the amount of time you exercise over several days or weeks depending on your condition. This might mean swimming longer distances or walking more briskly. Even the smallest of changes can make a big difference.

Flexibility Training – How To Improve Your Flexibility

Flexibility training can be very beneficial to individuals with CKD because fatigue can often lead to very little movement. After awhile, decreased movement can cause muscles to become tight. This can lead a decreased range of motion and even pain. Over time, it can also cause damage to muscles, joints, and bones. However, by stretching your tight muscles regularly you can help maintain your body's range of motion. Stretching and improving your body's flexibility can also improve your stride and balance and, by giving your muscles regular movement, increase your coordination. If you want to minimize your risk for injury and continue to be able to perform your daily activities and stay active then you must be able to continue to preserve your range of motion and your flexibility.

Regular physical activity and stretching exercises will improve your flexibility and prevent stiffness in your muscles. You should strive to do these along with any resistance training that you do. These can be done as warm-up exercises or as cool-down exercises. Holding your muscles in different positions for at least 30 seconds will help you get the most benefit from stretching them.

Tai Chi

Tai Chi is a slow, elegant, and flowing form of exercising. You don't need any special type of clothing or shoes. It almost appears like dancing and sometimes the moves appear undetectable. It is a centuries-old Chinese practice and deeply rooted in Chinese meditation, medicine, and martial arts. Tai chi combines mental awareness with slow, controlled movements in order to focus the mind, challenge the body, and improve the flow of "chi," the life energy that sustains health.

The exercises are simple and calming. However, because the exercises depend on fluidity, form, and movement (like a dance) it's difficult to list specific exercises individually. Finding a community center that offers Tai Chi can be a great way to participate with others in this calming and invigorating form of exercising that's beneficial not only for the body but the mind as well.

Tai Chi Pouring

A good beginning exercise is tai chi pouring. In this exercise you keep your feet flat on the floor, parallel, shoulder-width apart. Slowly pour your weight to your right side, allowing it to become full and the left empty. Hold for a few seconds. Pour your weight back to center. Now, gently pour your weight to the left side. Continue pouring from side to side, breathing naturally, for 2-3 minutes. This simple exercise can be done just about anywhere.

Yoga

Yoga can improve muscle tone, flexibility and balance. It can also help you relax and reduce stress levels. Research has shown that yoga has even been able to reduce symptoms of chronic pain, depression, and anxiety. Yoga can be done in studios under the direction of instructors. This might be something that you want to consider in the beginning, if you've never done yoga before. Or this can be done at home if you're a little more advanced. Below are a few examples of some traditional yoga poses.

Raised Arms Pose

This is a good stretch to do first thing in the morning. Inhale and bring your arms up over your head, but as you are focusing, keep your shoulders from moving away from your ears at the same time that you reach up through your fingertips. Your gaze can come up to the hands, which can be shoulder's width apart or palms touching.

Cat-Cow

Get on your mat on all fours with your hands directly below your shoulders and your knees below your hips. Distribute your weight between your hands and spread your fingers wide. Inhale and round your back, arching it up as you lower your chin to your chest. You should feel the stretch from your neck to your tailbone, like a cat. As you breathe out, lower your back down all the way to a scoop shape as you lift your head, and tilt it back. Repeat a few times to loosen your spine and open your chest.

Downward Facing Dog

In the downward-facing dog, your body makes an overturned V-shape (similar to the stretch that dogs do when they get up from a nap). Place both hands on the mat in front of you, palms down. Your hands should be somewhat in front of your shoulders. Place your knees on the ground straight under your hips. Breathe out as you lift your knees off the ground and lift your buttocks and hips toward the ceiling. Push the top of your thighs back and stretch your heels down toward the floor. Keep your head down between your upper arms and in line with them, not hanging down. Look at your stomach. You want to create a long straight spine. Hold the position for 5 to 10 breaths.

5 Ways to Increase Your Flexibility

1. Start out with slow stretches, work your way to full stretches, and then wind back down again with slow stretches in a workout.
2. Make sure you stretch every day, even on days when you're not working out.
3. Practice good posture.
4. Stay hydrated.
5. Make sure you feel the strain in your muscles. It should pull without hurting.

Planning An Exercise Program

Before you embark upon an exercise program, it's important to get your doctor's ok and to have a plan. Ensure that you plan a program that is proper for your comfort and health levels to maximize your efforts. Even for individuals suffering from end-stage renal disease, regular exercise can be extremely beneficial. It is advantageous that an exercise program be designed to fit your own physical abilities to eliminate the possibility of over-exerting yourself or exercising to the point of exhaustion.

Knowing Your Limits

Knowing the intensity level of your exercise can be tricky. Without knowing your exercise capacity, it can be challenging to know how much is "too much." Still, there are some guidelines that you might want to take into consideration.

For instance, you shouldn't be breathing so hard that you're unable to talk to someone when you are exercising. You should also feel completely "normal" within an hour after exercising; meaning that your heart rate and breathing are back to normal rates and your energy is back on track. In addition, you should feel a good kind of sore. You shouldn't feel so achy that you're unable to exercise again on the next day. If you're too sore, then you might want to bring it down a notch, or it could also mean that you're not warming up enough. You should start each session out slowly, ensuring that you're adequately warming up. Pick your pace up and then slowly wind down again before you finish.

Avoid exercising:

- Right after you've eaten a large meal
- If it's really hot
- Less than an hour before bedtime

- If you're really tired
- If you have an irregular heartbeat
- If you feel sick
- If your leg is cramping
- If you feel light headed
- If you have a fever

Integrating Exercise Into Your Lifestyle

In the beginning, you should start working out slowly. Work toward 30 minutes per session. You might find that you must gradually build toward this level. Ideally, you will exercise at least 20-30 minutes three days per week. After a while, you might find that you are able to exercise for as long as 45-60 minutes at a time.

Although you're aiming for three days per week, these don't have to be consecutive days. It's good to give your body the chance to recuperate and rest in between days when you're not exercising. Try to aim for non-consecutive days, such as, Monday, Wednesday and Friday. (You can do cardio daily and strength training every other day)

The types of exercises that you choose can really make a difference in the success of your overall exercise program. Continuous activity, such as walking or swimming, will allow you to continuously move large muscle groups. This is one of the reasons why aerobic exercise is recommended for individuals with chronic kidney disease.

You might also find that low-level strengthening exercises are beneficial as part of your exercise program. When you use low weights and high repetitions, and avoid heavy lifting, you can strengthen your muscles without over-exerting yourself.

Your Diet and Exercise Program

Even when you're on an exercise program, you must still continue to abide by any dietary restrictions that you ordinarily follow unless otherwise dictated by your physician. Even regular exercise doesn't give you permission to eat foods that are restricted from your chronic kidney disease diet.

Your chronic kidney disease diet and exercise program should work together, not replace one another. Together, they should be able to help ensure that you live a healthier lifestyle and offer you a better quality of life. By following a plan, you have more control over your health and the choices you make. Following one doesn't mean you're able to ignore the other. However, if you do notice an increase in your appetite after starting an exercise program then you should discuss this with your doctor or your renal dietitian. They will be able to help you ensure your calorie intake is sufficient.

If you consume restricted foods it can jeopardize your health and could cause problems, especially if you're on dialysis. You should always ask your physician and/or renal dietitian about eating foods that aren't specified in your early or late stage kidney diet. Sometimes certain foods are limited because they contain a lot of sugar, potassium, fat, sodium or phosphorus and these can be harmful. Depending on which stage of chronic kidney disease you are in, you might need to replace any lost fluids.

You may need to monitor your urine output. If you're urinating less and sweating more, it may be necessary to increase your fluid intake. However, before you make any changes on your own, discuss it with your doctor. It might take awhile to find the right balance that's healthy for you.

The Exercise Program

Since each individual's health and fitness levels, motivation and time constraints are going to vary, there aren't any general guidelines that apply to all individuals with renal disease. When planning your exercise program, however, you are generally going to be looking at the type of exercises, frequency, duration, and intensity. You might also be considering the setting, too.

Type of Exercises

The type of exercises that you do can vary and will depend on your range of motion, endurance, and what you enjoy doing. You should do a variety of aerobic activity, which increases your rate and gets your blood pumping, and resistance training, which strengthens your muscles.

Continuous exercises are ideal. These are also good for those who experience joint pain and include such exercises are walking, swimming, aerobic dancing, and bicycling. This type of exercising is also good because it can be started out at a slower pace and gradually increased over a period of time as endurance is built up.

Exercise Examples:

Strengthening exercises:

1. Standing up and sitting down several times: a quick workout that exercises your calves and thigh muscles
2. Rising up and down on your toes: strengthens your toes, ankles, and calves using your own bodyweight
3. Stepping up and down off a step: a good workout for your entire leg, especially your calves and thighs (but also your glutes). If you can, try going up and down an entire staircase as many times as possible in a day.

4. Lifting weights: strengthens biceps and triceps. They don't have to be heavy weights. Start out with a little resistance, even something small (like a can of soup). Gradually work your way up 5 pounds or more if you can.
5. Leg Lifts: leg lifts not only strengthen leg muscles but also work abdominal muscles, including obliques, too.
6. Arm Circles: arm circles, which include holding your arms out to your side and slowly moving them in measured circles, help build stamina and muscles. The longer you can do them without tiring out, the more strength and endurance you can build.

Cardiovascular exercises:

1. Walking: walking can be done inside (indoor tracks, shopping centers, etc.) or outside and either alone or with groups. It can also be done at any pace you feel comfortable thus, making it extremely adaptable.
2. Cycling: cycling is an extremely versatile cardiovascular activity. With spinning classes becoming increasingly popular, it's also possible to cycle indoors with other people in a more social setting these days as well.
3. Swimming: swimming is a cardiovascular activity that works out the entire body and is gentle on the joints which is good for those who also suffer from chronic pain or inflammation. It can be enjoyed year round if you have access to an indoor swimming pool.
4. Dancing: there are many forms of dancing available right now, from the energetic zumba to ballroom dancing, aerobics, adult ballet, and even adult-oriented Iris step dancing classes that some community centers offer.
5. Jogging: if you enjoy jogging then ensure you have the right kind of shoes in order to cut down on potential back and foot

problems. Check around your neighborhood to see if there are any local running groups if you don't want to jog alone.

6. Water aerobics/ water walking: as previously mentioned, water sports are easy on the joints and offer a lot of resistance.

7. Elliptical machines: elliptical machines can be enjoyed in the gym or in your own home if you prefer to work out in the privacy of your house. These work several key muscle groups in your body and have a variety of settings.

Chair exercises:

1. If you're extremely mobility-limited then there are still some activities that you can enjoy from your sofa or your chair. These can help strengthen your arms and your legs and help increase your flexibility and strength in these areas:

2. Wrap a lightweight resistance band under your chair (or sofa) and carry out quick resistance exercises, such as chest presses, for a count of one second up and two seconds down. Try a number of different exercises to start, with 5 to 10 reps per exercise. Gradually increase the number of exercises, reps, and total workout time as your endurance improves.

3. Attach resistance bands to furniture, a doorknob, or your chair. Use these for pull-downs, shoulder rotations, and arm and leg-extensions.

4. Sit tall with the abs in and hold a full water bottle in your left hand. Lift the bottle up to shoulder level, pause, and then continue lifting all the way up over your head. When your arm is next to your ear, bend your elbow, taking the water bottle behind you and contracting your triceps. Straighten the arm and lower down, repeating for 10 reps on each arm. Increase your reps as your strength increases.

Frequency

How often you exercise is generally the next thing that you will be looking at. Most studies show that to get the most benefits out of an exercise program you should aim at working out at least 3-5 times per week every other day. You can do cardio exercise on consecutive days, if you would like, and exercising every day is ok too once your body is used to it. Just be careful of your recover time.

Duration

For the actual working out period, you will probably aim for at least 30 minutes on most days. However, you should try to factor in at least several minutes of stretching and warming up. At the end of every workout period, some time should be spent cooling down as well. When you first start out, begin at a level that is suitable for you, e.g. 5 minutes per session. From there, steadily build up the duration of each session by adding 1 or 2 minutes each week. About 30 minutes per session is a good level to aspire for, though you may feel like exercising even longer.

Even a little bit of activity every day is better than no activity at all. If you're unable to exercise every day then rearranging your schedule to fit in some form of physical activity is desirable. This might mean taking the stairs instead of the elevator or walking around the block. It might even mean vacuuming the living room, stretching for 10-15 minutes before bed, or doing half an hour of chair exercises in front of the television before you go to bed at night. Continuing to stay mobile and active is the important part, even when you are unable to fit in an entire exercise session.

Intensity

Exercise intensity depends on your individual capacity. Generally speaking, you should feel totally recovered within an hour of exercising and shouldn't feel so much discomfort that you are unable to exercise the next day. Every session should begin with a slow warm up, rise to a comfortable level, and then slow down again before finishing.

Over time you will gradually be able to build up endurance and stamina. You should, in your strength training, feel a pull. However, it shouldn't hurt. If you feel pain then you're doing too much. Although you might feel uncomfortable, exercising should never hurt. If you feel short of breath or unable to talk, or breathe, or catch your breath, or that you're sweating so much that you feel dehydrated then you are overdoing it. If your exercise session is so intense that you're unable to work out the next day then you need to scale it back and reevaluate the way you are working out.

Setting

Not every workout environment is ideal for every person. Some people work out very well in a gym or health club. Others do a lot better in the privacy of their own home. Some people work out better when they have the support of other people around. Others feel too self-conscious when others around and they're too embarrassed when they feel like others are watching them. Some people like exercising with strength training equipment and machines such as weight machines and treadmills. Others prefer to ride bikes on trails and take walks outside. The important thing is to find what works for you.

You might find that as you get more comfortable working out in one setting that you want to try branching out into something else. For instance, you may start out working out at home. Once you feel comfortable after a few weeks or months in your home, you might decide to give the gym a try. Perhaps you may notice that the local gym is offering a discount for a month and decide to try it out to see how you like it.

It's okay to change your mind!

You shouldn't be surprised if, after you become more confident with yourself, your feelings change about how you want to proceed in the future. As you begin exercising you might also meet new people and make new friends. This may also influence how you proceed in the future. You could be invited, for instance, to join a new exercise group, such as a jogging group or cycling group. New opportunities might present themselves to you that you wouldn't have seen in the past. By keeping yourself open to possibilities you can really expand your horizons.

Walking with Chronic Kidney Disease

Walking is one of the best exercises when it comes to getting up and moving with chronic kidney disease. It moves the large muscle groups repetitively and you can do it inside or outside, and fast or slow. Walking can be a social activity, something that you can get your family or friends to do with you. It allows you to remain active and can help you improve your overall health. A few of the benefits of walking include:

- Good blood circulation

- Blood pressure control

- Stress relief

- Stronger muscles

- Weight control

Remember, it's important to stay hydrated while you are walking. But it's also important for CKD patients to stay within their prescribed fluid limits if you have them. You should consult your healthcare team about how to remain hydrated while walking and still manage your fluid intake. In addition, check the labels on any of your water bottles and sports drinks since a lot of the brands have extra potassium or phosphorus, something that kidney disease patients need to know.

Joining A Group

There are lots of different groups available for support for those with chronic kidney disease and many of these have excellent exercise programs available. For instance, check with your local senior citizens center, or your YMCA. Many of these have regular exercise groups or recreational groups that meet regularly and some of these might be free or have a nominal fee. Working out with others who have similar interests or medical conditions might offer the support that you need to meet the goals that you have set for yourself.

Barriers to Exercising

Even knowing all the benefits and advantages that exercising can have in your overall health, there can still be barriers to finding ways to working a regular program into your lifestyle. Overcoming these barriers might be challenging, but it's important to figure out a way to make it possible in order to realize the best possible quality of life.

Common Barriers

1. Not enough time.

Finding time in your schedule to exercise can be difficult, especially if you also work or have other obligations. You might have to be creative to find extra time in your day to exercise. If you don't have time to go to a gym then you can find other opportunities to work out, even if it means using non-traditional methods to exercise. This could mean doing things such as:

- Walking instead of driving when you can
- Taking the stairs instead of the elevator
- Taking a brisk walk around the block every night after supper
- Getting up an extra 30 minutes every morning to exercise in your living room with a video
- Squeezing in an extra work out session every Saturday or Sunday morning

2. You feel self-conscious

Some people find the idea of exercising in front of others makes them feel self-conscious. They worry about how they look when they are working out and how they appear in their exercise clothes. The fact is, most people are not actually looking at other people. Instead, they're concentrating on performing the moves correctly themselves. Instead of focusing on how others are perceiving you, concentrate on the favor you're doing for your health. If you still find that you feel too self-conscious then consider investing in some inexpensive workout equipment for home, like a stationary bike. Perhaps you could look at garage sales for stationary bikes, elliptical machines, or weights. Try to go to a gym early in the morning or after lunch when others are less likely to be there.

3. You feel too tired

As previously mentioned, feeling too tried to exercise can actually be a vicious inactivity cycle. Without some form of regular activity you will find that you don't have the energy to exercise at all and you'll continue to feel tired. For extra boosts of energy throughout the day, try the following:

- Try sticking to a regular sleeping schedule so that you're getting ample sleep at night. Aim for at least 8 hours of solid sleep.
- Follow your dietitian's recommendations as far as your dietary plan goes, and don't skip meals.
- If you get too tired during the day, take a short nap, but don't sleep for more than an hour or else you might not be able to sleep at night.
- Always cool down after exercising so that your muscles have the chance to relax.
- Exercise in the morning or afternoon instead of in the evening.

4. You don't feel athletic

Some people have never really felt athletic. They didn't excel at sports in school and have never before joined a gym. They don't even know where to start when it comes to exercising. However, you don't have to possess a natural athletic ability to enjoy physical activity. When you're trying to increase your endurance and improve your flexibility, start simple and forget about competing with the other athletes you might see at the gym. Instead, keep your exercises easy and try to stick with things that are basic, like walks. You can also work with a team of others and maybe join up with friends who also want to work out regularly. Perhaps meet with a group of likeminded individuals (maybe even others with CKD or others with chronic conditions) and begin walking around the neighborhood together or meeting several times a week to go swimming.

5. You can't afford the fees

Health club fees and gym memberships can be expensive. However, you don't have to join these pricey places in order to get the benefits of regular exercise. There are alternatives that can be just as advantageous. Consider the following:

- **Do resistance training at home.** Inexpensive resistance bands, instead of weights, can be used at home. You can also start out with soup cans, plastic milk jugs with sand, or anything else with a little bit of weight to them. Squats and push-ups can be used with your own body weight for resistance training.
- **Use videos.** Videos can be watched online, bought at garage sales, or even checked out from the library. Use them alone or watch them with a friend if you want to work out with the support of someone else. You might try the Senior Citizen's center. And of course, there is always You Tube which has good exercise videos on it. There are lots of great places to find free videos. You might even consider starting a video exchange club with a group of friends.
- **Try your community center.** There are often exercise classes offered through a local recreation department or community centers. These classes are usually offered at nominal costs and are much cheaper than gym memberships

and give you the opportunity to work out with other members of the community.

Setting Goals

Setting goals in your exercising endeavors can help you achieve expectations that aren't as overwhelming as they might seem. You want your goals to be small and realistic because if your bar is set too high, you might give up too quickly-maybe before you really get started.

Make gaining endurance one of your goals. For instance, start out with taking yourself for a walk around your block every afternoon. If you don't feel too tired after that then after a week move up to going twice around your block. Gradually increase the amount of activity that you are doing.

Listen to your body when you are setting your goals. This might mean working with your body and not against it. There might be certain times of the day when you naturally have more energy. If you are naturally more energetic in the mornings then set your alarm for thirty minutes earlier than usual. Use that time to do some stretches.

Making a Commitment

Making a commitment and planning on carrying through with your goal to exercise is important. Although you might not be able to see your results in the beginning, but your body will be able to feel them and that's important. If it helps, make a schedule and stick to it. That might mean that you have to actually create a calendar, post it somewhere visible in your home or office, and pencil in the days and times that you're going to exercise. Your exercise plan should be as important as keeping your doctors' appointments and is considered a necessary part of your treatment plan. By considering them essential to your overall health, you'll be more likely to keep up with your exercise regimen.

Managing Your Health While You Exercise

It is important to talk to your doctor before you start any kind of physical activity program. Your doctor should be able to tell you what exercises are best for you or any limitations you might have since they will have a good understanding of your current stage of kidney disease and treatment. More than likely, your doctor will be pleased that you're asking about exercise. They might even be able to refer you to a physical therapist for extra help. A physical therapist can help monitor your progress and activity level.

A lot of people on dialysis have additional medical concerns such as heart disease or diabetes. These may affect your stamina or capacity to exercise. This is why it's important to start out slowly, and then steadily work up to heavier weights or longer times.

If you have diabetes then you might need to watch your sugar levels since exercise cause your blood sugar levels to fall. This might tell you when you need to adjust your medication. Of course, you should never do this without first talking to your doctor.

It's normal to feel tired and even a little short of breath afterward exercise, especially in the beginning. It's also natural to have aching muscles when you are finished. You should never exercise to the point of collapse. If you experience any symptoms such as chest pain, unexpected shortness of breath, or relentless muscular or joint pain then you should stop exercising and talk to your doctor.

Next Steps

1. Once you've made the decision to start an exercise program the first thing you really need to do to is talk to your doctor. He or she will be able to set you on the right path. They will probably be supportive of your decision and maybe even be able to point you in the right direction as far as what health club recommendations or group memberships might be available. They will also be able to let you know if there are any limitations that might be individual to you and your own medical conditions. Remember that any exercising that you do will not supersede any dietary restrictions that you might already possess.

2. Preferably, your exercise program will be incorporated into your regular daily routine and, in time, will become easy and even pleasurable. It should become a part of your everyday life and in no time at all you'll become used to it and will start seeing the positive effects of it.

3. Keep in mind that you should always talk to your medical team before you start doing anything different in regards to your health. You might need to be evaluated if there are any changes, especially in regards to your fluid intake. It's important for you to remain as healthy as possible. Your exercise program can be treated as part of your overall healthcare plan and, if done properly, can hopefully work to offer you a better quality of life so that you can enjoy independence and the active, happy life you deserve.

Go to
www.renaldiethq.com/go/
exercise and sign up for
the mailing list to
receive a book of 25
Low Impact Exercises
for people with CKD
that are great for you
to do.

Other Titles By Mathea Ford:

Mathea Ford, Author Page (all books):

http://www.amazon.com/Mathea-Ford/e/B008E1E7IS/

The Kidney Friendly Diet Cookbook

http://www.amazon.com/Kidney-Friendly-Diet-Cookbook-PreDialysis-ebook/dp/B00BC7BGPI/

Create Your Own Kidney Diet Plan

http://www.amazon.com/Create-Your-Kidney-Diet-Plan-ebook/dp/B009PSN3R0/

Living with Chronic Kidney Disease - Pre-Dialysis

http://www.amazon.com/Living-Chronic-Kidney-Disease-Pre-Dialysis-ebook/dp/B008D8RSAQ/

Eating a Pre-Dialysis Kidney Diet - Calories, Carbohydrates, Fat & Protein, Secrets To Avoid Dialysis

http://www.amazon.com/Eating-Pre-Dialysis-Kidney-Diet-Carbohydrates-ebook/dp/B00DU2JCHM/

Eating a Pre-Dialysis Kidney Diet - Sodium, Potassium, Phosphorus and Fluids, A Kidney Disease Solution

http://www.amazon.com/Eating-Pre-Dialysis-Kidney-Diet-Phosphorus-ebook/dp/B00E2U8VMS/

Eating Out On a Kidney Diet: Pre-dialysis and Diabetes: Ways To Enjoy Your Favorite Foods

http://www.amazon.com/Eating-Out-Kidney-Diet-Pre-dialysis/dp/0615928781/

Kidney Disease: Common Labs and Medical Terminology: The Patient's Perspective

http://www.amazon.com/Kidney-Disease-Terminology-Perspective-Pre-Dialysis/dp/0615931804/

Dialysis: Treatment Options for the Progression to End Stage Renal Disease

http://www.amazon.com/Dialysis-Treatment-Options-Progression-Disease/dp/0615932258/

Mindful Eating For A Pre-Dialysis Kidney Diet: Healthy Attitudes Toward Food and Life

http://www.amazon.com/Mindful-Eating-Pre-Dialysis-Kidney-Diet/dp/0615933475/

The Emotional Challenges Of Coping with Chronic Kidney Disease

http://www.amazon.com/Emotional-Challenges-Chronic-Disease-Dialysis-ebook/dp/B00H6SYQG8/

www.ingramcontent.com/pod-product-compliance
Lightning Source LLC
Chambersburg PA
CBHW060526280326
41933CB00014B/3104